AF207011

BECOME A
RESPIRATORY THERAPIST

by Mike Downs

BrightPoint Press

San Diego, CA

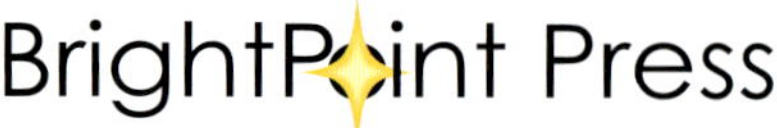

© 2025 BrightPoint Press
an imprint of ReferencePoint Press, Inc.
Printed in the United States

For more information, contact:
BrightPoint Press
PO Box 27779
San Diego, CA 92198
www.BrightPointPress.com

LIBRARY OF CONGRESS CATALOGING-IN-PUBLICATION DATA

Names: Downs, Mike, author.
Title: Become a respiratory therapist / by Mike Downs.
Description: San Diego, CA: BrightPoint, [2025] | Series: Skilled and vocational trades | Includes bibliographical references and index. | Audience: Grades 7-9
Identifiers: LCCN 2024001068 (print) | LCCN 2024001069 (eBook) | ISBN 9781678209001 (hardcover) | ISBN 9781678209018 (eBook)
Subjects: LCSH: Respiratory therapists--Vocational guidance--Juvenile literature.
Classification: LCC RM161.D696 2025 (print) | LCC RM161 (eBook) | DDC 615.8/2023--dc23/eng/20240124
LC record available at https://lccn.loc.gov/2024001068
LC eBook record available at https://lccn.loc.gov/2024001069

CONTENTS

AT A GLANCE

- Respiratory therapists help people who have trouble breathing. They help everyone from young babies to seniors.

- A respiratory therapist attends every emergency at a hospital. Many emergency patients have trouble breathing.

- Most respiratory therapists work in large hospitals. Some respiratory therapists can also work in home care or sleep labs. They work in pulmonary clinics, and they sell ventilator equipment.

- Respiratory therapy training takes about 3 years. Some colleges have started 2-year programs.

- Respiratory therapists helped respond to the COVID-19 pandemic. Many COVID-19 patients need help breathing.

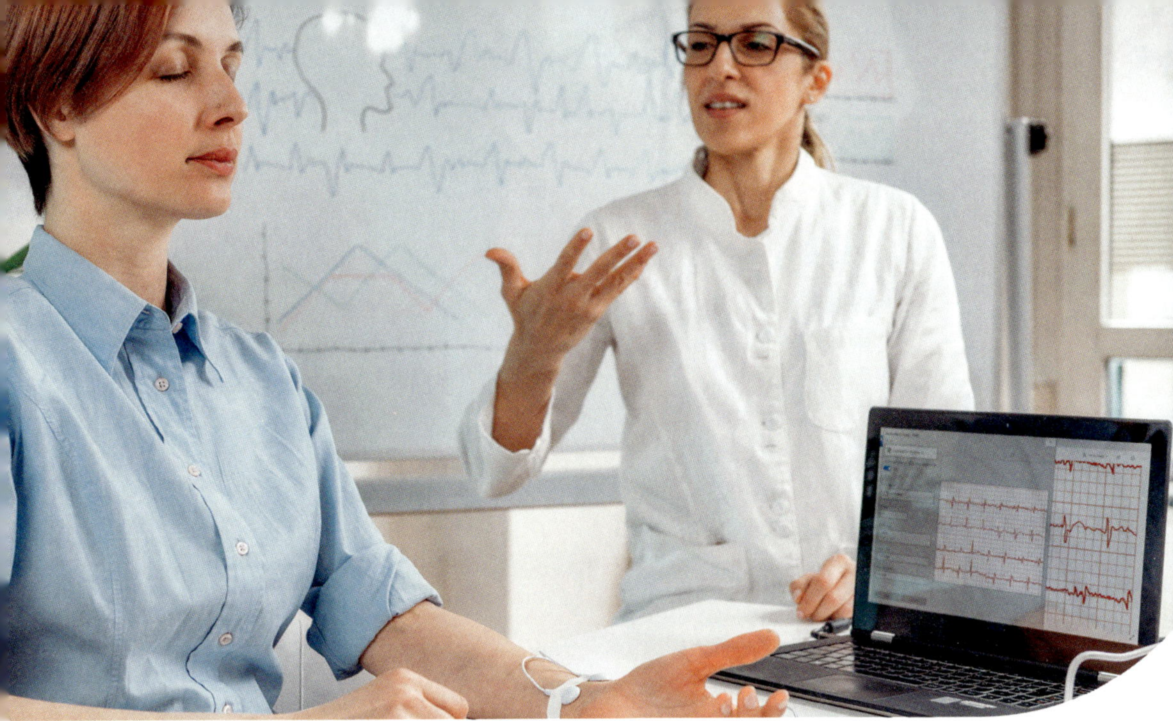

- Some respiratory therapists specialize in lung function tests. These tests measure how well a person can breathe.

- Environmental factors are making breathing issues worse around the world. This will increase the need for respiratory therapists.

- The American Association for Respiratory Care (AARC) is creating a new career path. It is called Advanced Practice Respiratory Therapist (APRT).

WHY BECOME A RESPIRATORY THERAPIST?

Misty Carlson explained, "There is nothing more important than breathing!"[1] She was talking about her daughter, Kylee. Kylee was born early and had trouble breathing. A respiratory therapist (RT) helped. The RT suctioned **mucus** out of Kylee's throat. She used a machine to give her more oxygen. The RT helped Kylee breathe.

Respiratory therapists use suction devices to remove mucus from babies' noses and throats.

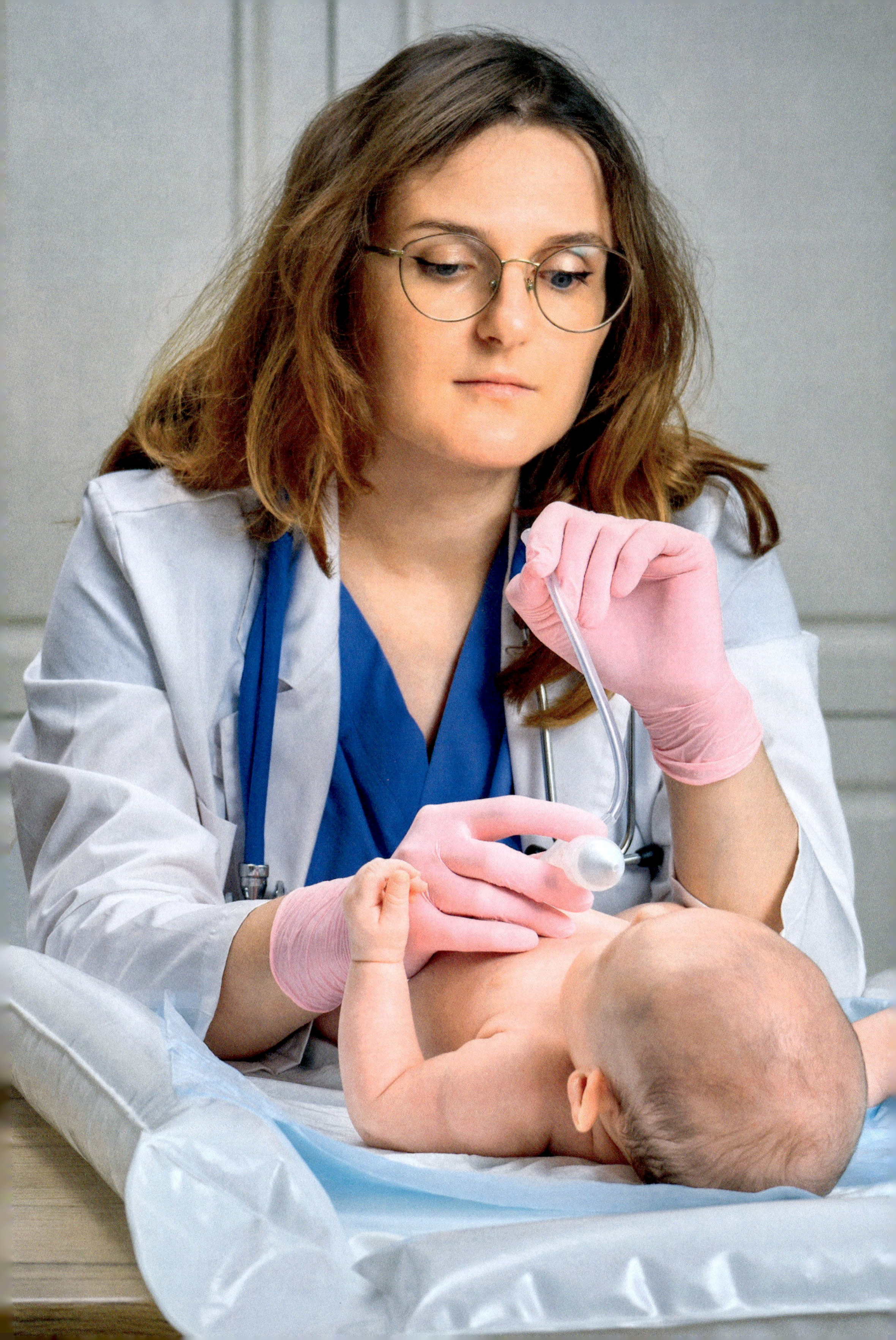

Misty took Kylee home from the hospital.
But as she grew up, Kylee still had trouble
breathing. RTs came to Misty's house to
help. They gave Kylee treatments. They
taught her how to get more air when
breathing. They showed her how to use
medications. Misty watched the RTs
work. She wanted to help other people
breathe, too.

Misty enrolled at Daytona State
College in Florida. She graduated with
an associate's degree in applied science.
She went to work at Halifax Hospital.
There she learned more about helping
people breathe. She went back to school
to earn a master's degree. She became
the clinical coordinator at Daytona State
College. "Our field is expanding," she said.

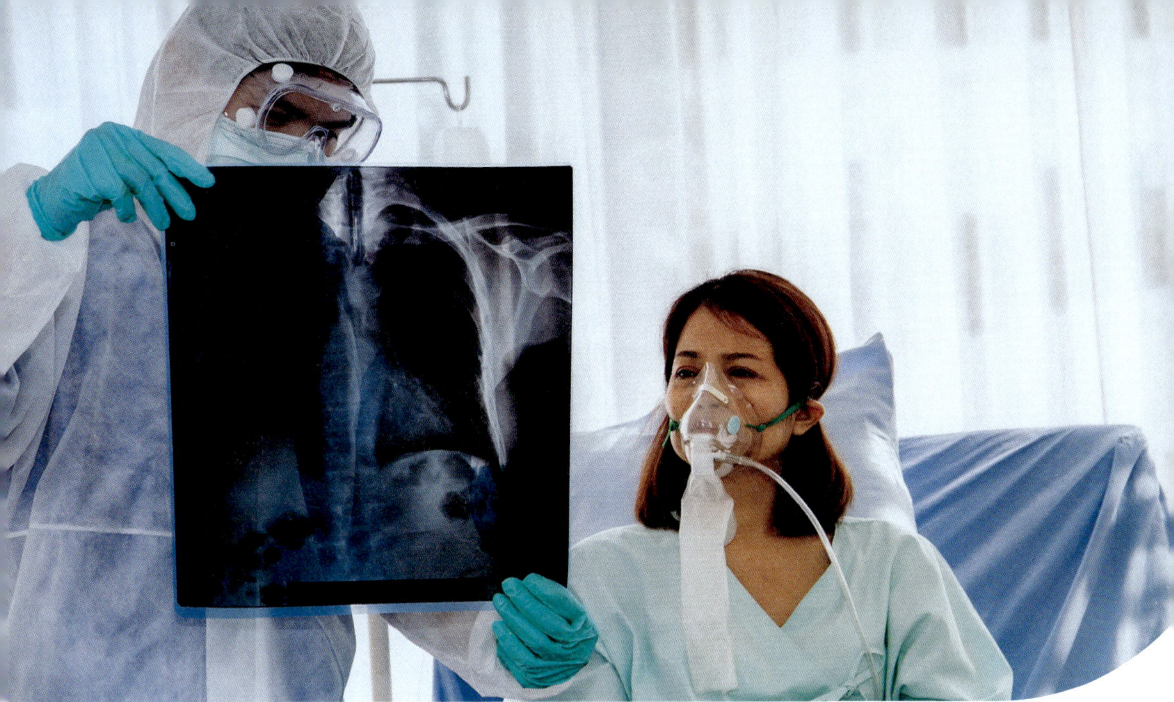

"We're there all the way from that first breath, until people die."[2]

WHAT IS A RESPIRATORY THERAPIST?

Respiratory therapists help people breathe in many different ways. They might use medication. In some cases they teach breathing skills. Other times they might use a breathing machine.

RTs are needed in every part of a hospital. They are very important in the **neonatal** intensive care unit (NICU). Therapists also help in the emergency room. They help cancer patients and patients with heart problems.

RTs help anyone who has trouble breathing. They work in hospitals. They also work in labs, nursing homes, and clinics. Respiratory therapists might become supervisors, teachers, or researchers, too.

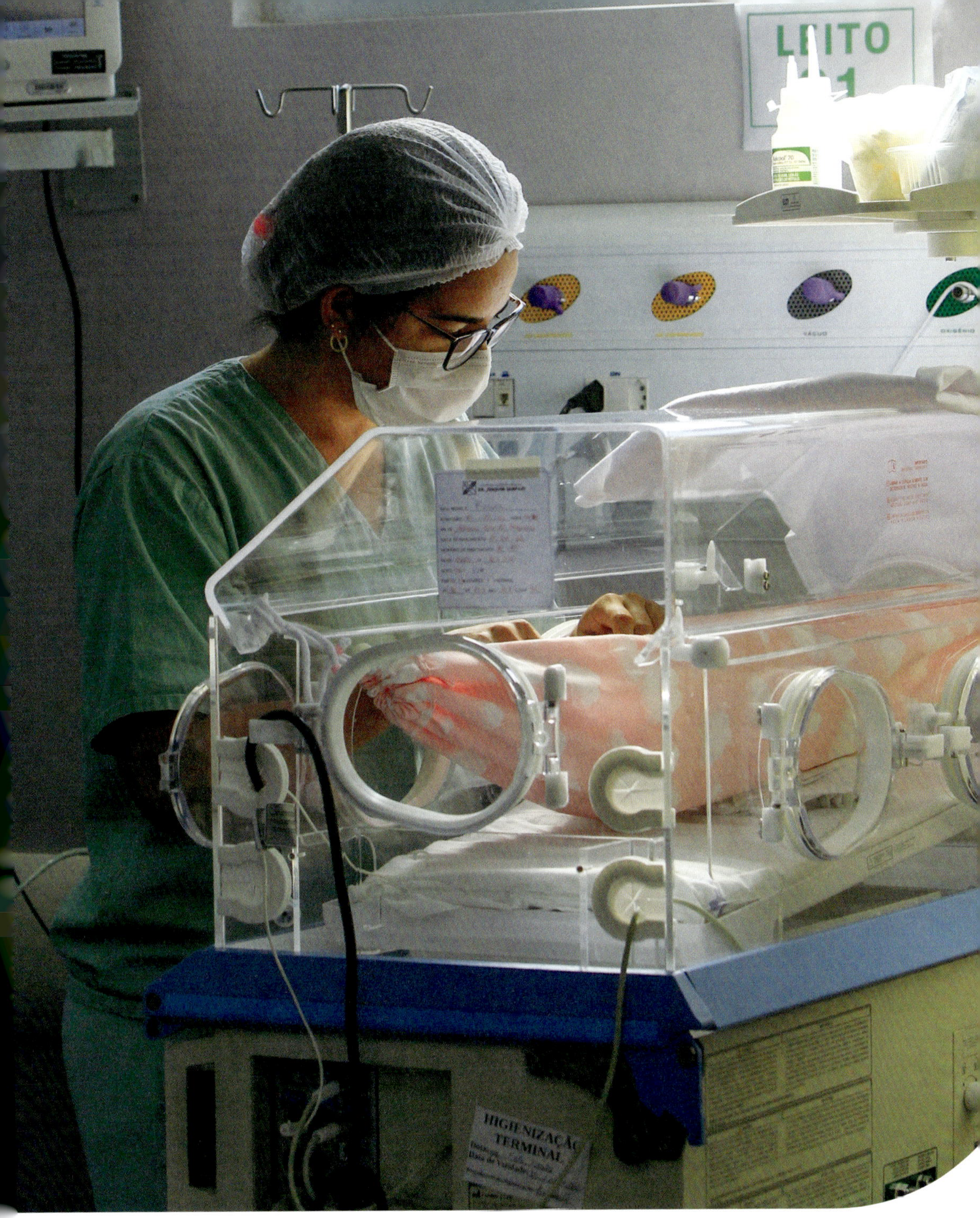

Babies in the NICU often have trouble breathing. They sleep in a covered, safe space called an incubator.

CHAPTER ONE

WHAT DOES A RESPIRATORY THERAPIST DO?

Respiratory therapists work in many areas of medicine. They help newborn babies and **COPD** patients. COPD is a disease that reduces airflow from the lungs. RTs work with heart and cancer patients. They help people with asthma or sleep problems. They help COVID-19 patients. RTs help anyone who has trouble breathing.

"It's always been a rewarding career," said Gina Ricard. "And I'm so happy I

A ventilator is one of the many tools RTs use to treat breathing issues.

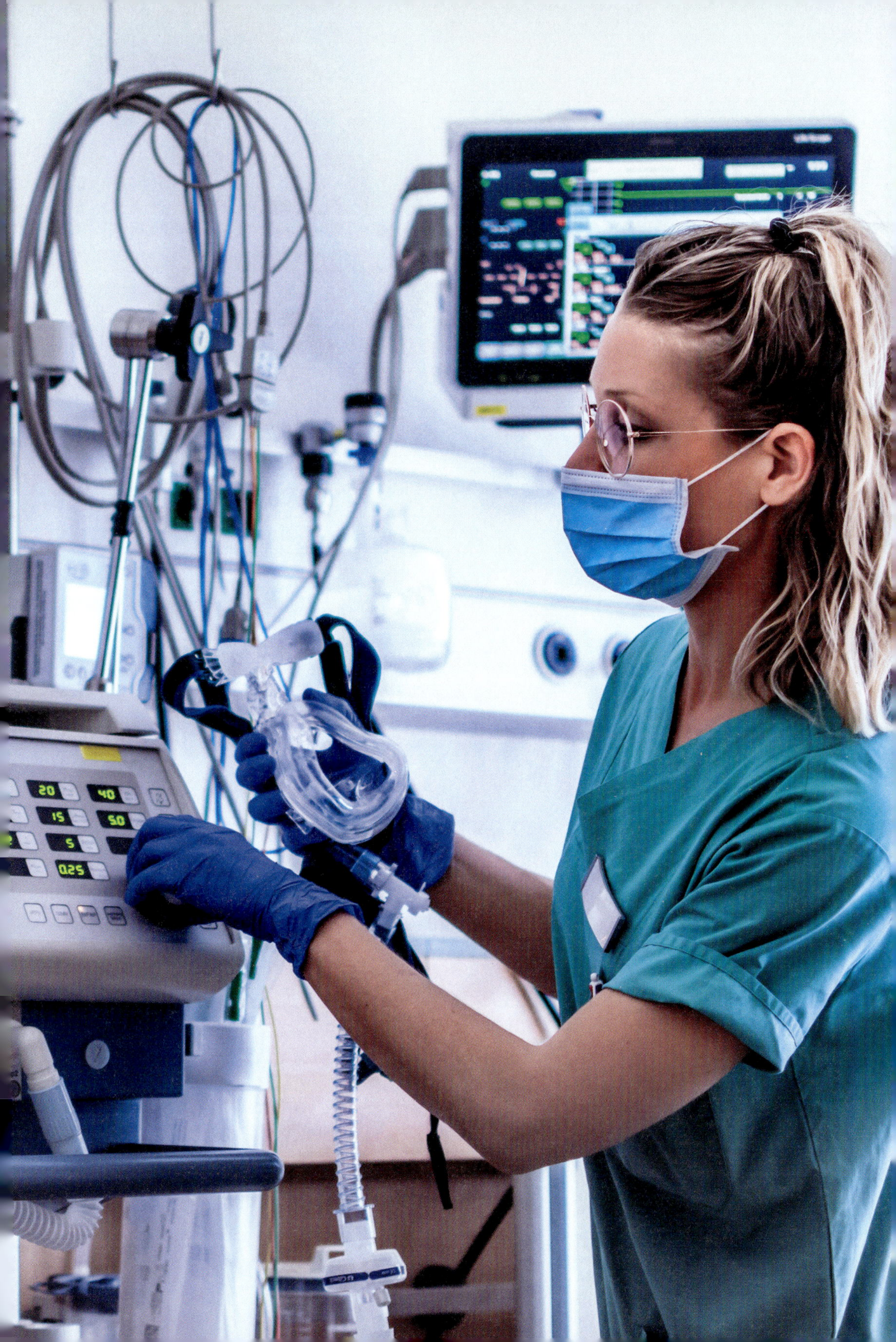

found it."[3] Ricard was an RT at SUNY Upstate Medical University. Then she decided to teach. This is one career path for respiratory therapists. Ricard worked in many roles over her career. She has worked with people who are dangerously sick. She has worked in home care, helping people at their homes. She has been a supervisor, a professor, and a program director. These are only a few of the many jobs respiratory therapists can do.

WORKING WITH BABIES

Some RTs enjoy working with newborns. They spend a lot of time in the NICU. This is where premature babies are born. These therapists help comfort moms. When the baby is born, therapists suction mucus

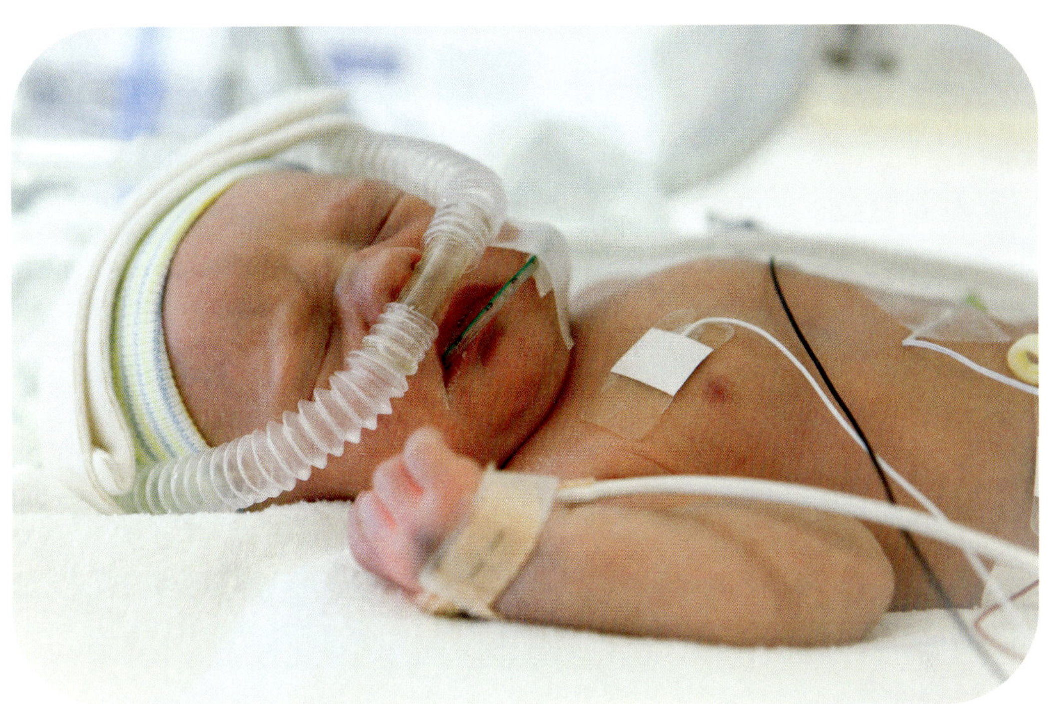

Babies who are born early sometimes need a CPAP machine to help them breathe.

from the baby's mouth. This helps to clear the airway. Sometimes babies have trouble breathing. The therapist might use a **CPAP machine**. This is a special breathing device. It pumps air into the baby's nose. Therapists do whatever they can to help the baby breathe.

RT Beth Howell helped one mom. The mom had given birth to quintuplets. That's five babies at once. An entire team of nurses, doctors, and RTs was needed. The team needed to have five breathing machines ready. They had to prepare.

"We rehearsed with baby dolls," explained Beth. After the **micro preemies** were born, the therapists used machines to help them breathe. All five survived. "It went so smooth," said Beth. "Forty years ago, these babies had no chance."[4]

BREATHING MACHINES

One part of an RT's job is to operate breathing machines. These are called ventilators. Patients need ventilators for different reasons. A patient might have **pneumonia**. This is an infection. It causes the lungs to fill with fluid. Some have COPD.

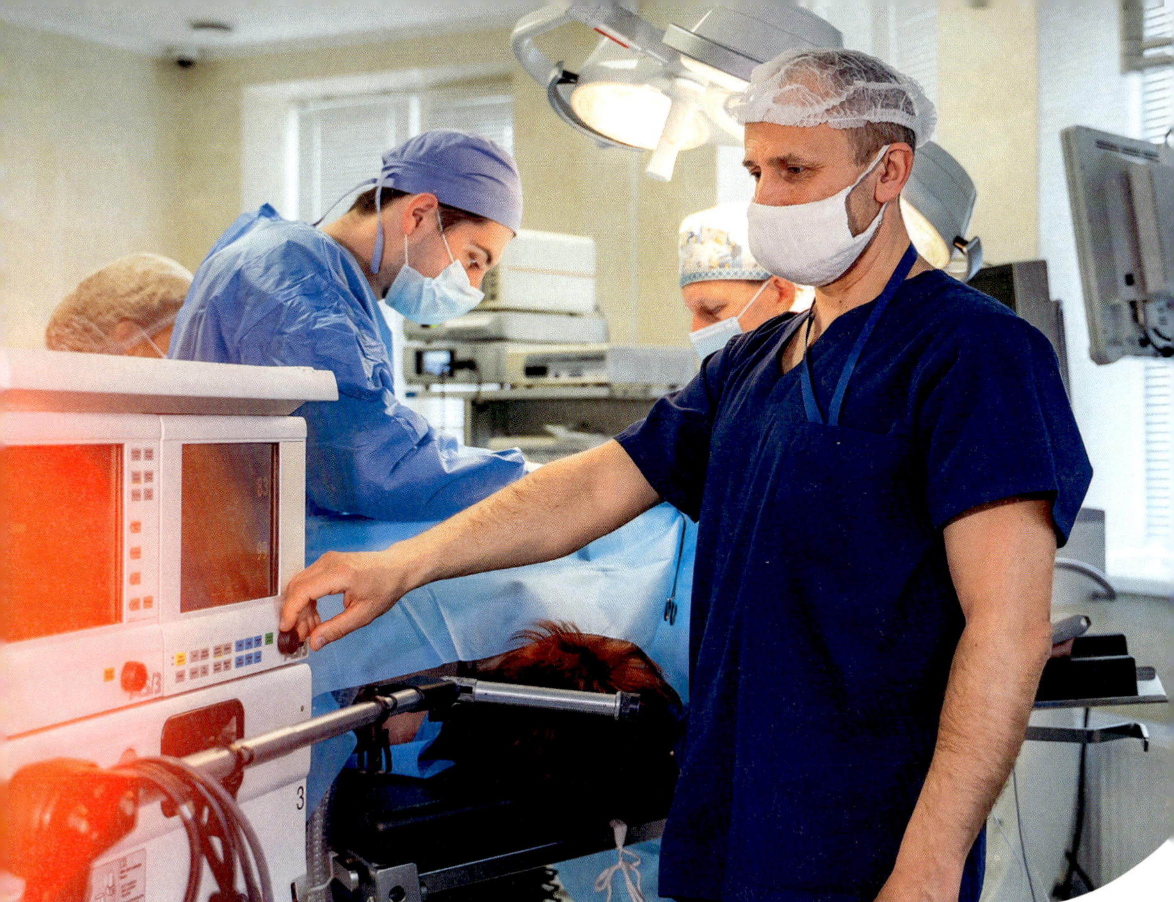

Part of an RTs job is to adjust the settings on ventilators to better meet patients' needs.

This can be caused by smoking or vaping. Asthma and other diseases can also cause breathing problems.

RTs use ventilators to help patients breathe. A ventilator moves air in and out of a person's lungs. Therapists must know how much air to pump in and out.

Different patients need different amounts. The RT sets the ventilator to pump the correct amount of air. The RT can also add more oxygen to the air. Ventilators pump this air into a mask. The patient wears this mask over their nose and mouth. Very ill patients need breathing tubes that go down into their throats.

Some patients have ventilators at home. RTs teach these patients how to use them. Other patients have CPAP machines at home. These machines help people sleep. RTs teach patients how to use CPAP machines. They also check to make sure the machines are working properly. If something is wrong with a machine, RTs figure out the problem. Sometimes they can fix the machines.

OTHER TASKS

RTs take blood samples as well. Most blood samples are taken from the veins on a patient's arm. These samples will show if the person has an infection or doesn't have enough red blood cells. Both of those conditions make it more difficult to breathe. Some RTs can do an arterial blood gas (ABG) test. RTs need extra training to do this test. They need to draw the blood from

Breathing Without Lungs

Some RTs operate extracorporeal membrane oxygenation (ECMO) machines. These machines take the blood out of the body. They add oxygen directly to the blood. Then they pump the blood back in. ECMO machines do the job of both the lungs and the heart. They are used for **critical care patients**.

an artery deep down in the patient's wrist. After they draw the blood, it is sent off for testing. This test shows whether a person's body is getting enough oxygen.

Some RTs travel with patients. Patients may need to move from one hospital to another. Some patients even return home

Patients continue to receive all the care they need while they are being transferred to a new facility.

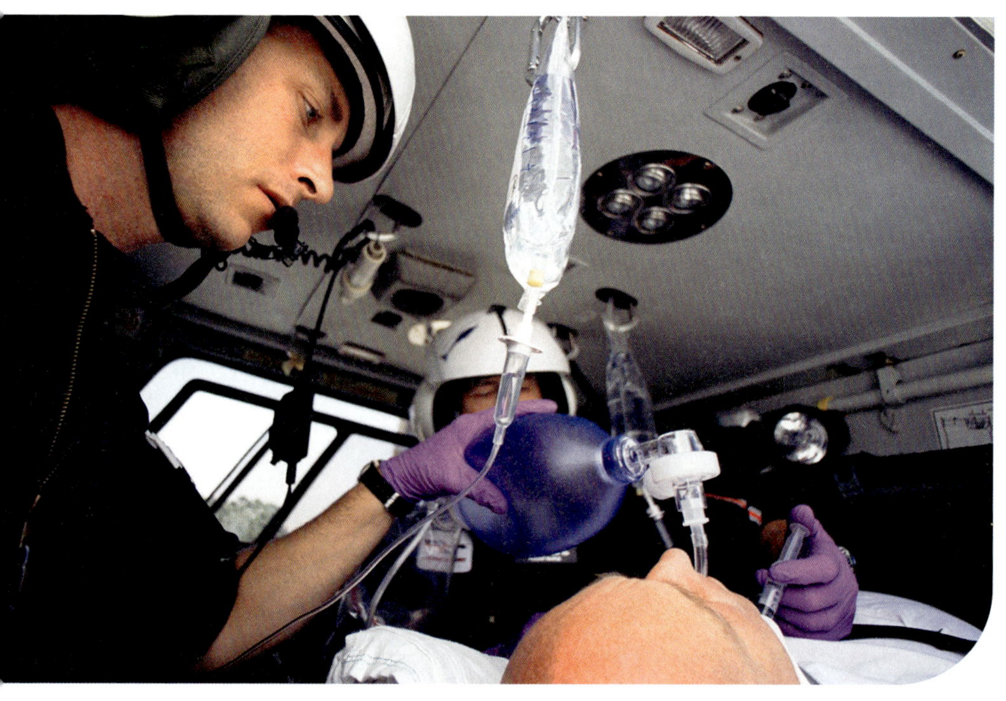

from other countries. An RT travels with
them. Therapists might travel with patients
on jets, helicopters, or ambulances. The RT
must assess the patient. Then they decide
how to help the patient breathe. During
travel the therapist makes sure the ventilator
is working correctly.

RTs also work in emergency rooms.
These therapists never know what breathing
problems they will treat each day. Patients
with many different health problems come
to the emergency room. RTs might treat
the victim of a car crash or a shooting.
They might help an injured baby. Or they
may save someone who overdosed on
drugs. When a patient is brought into an
emergency room, several people work
to help them. A paramedic might bring

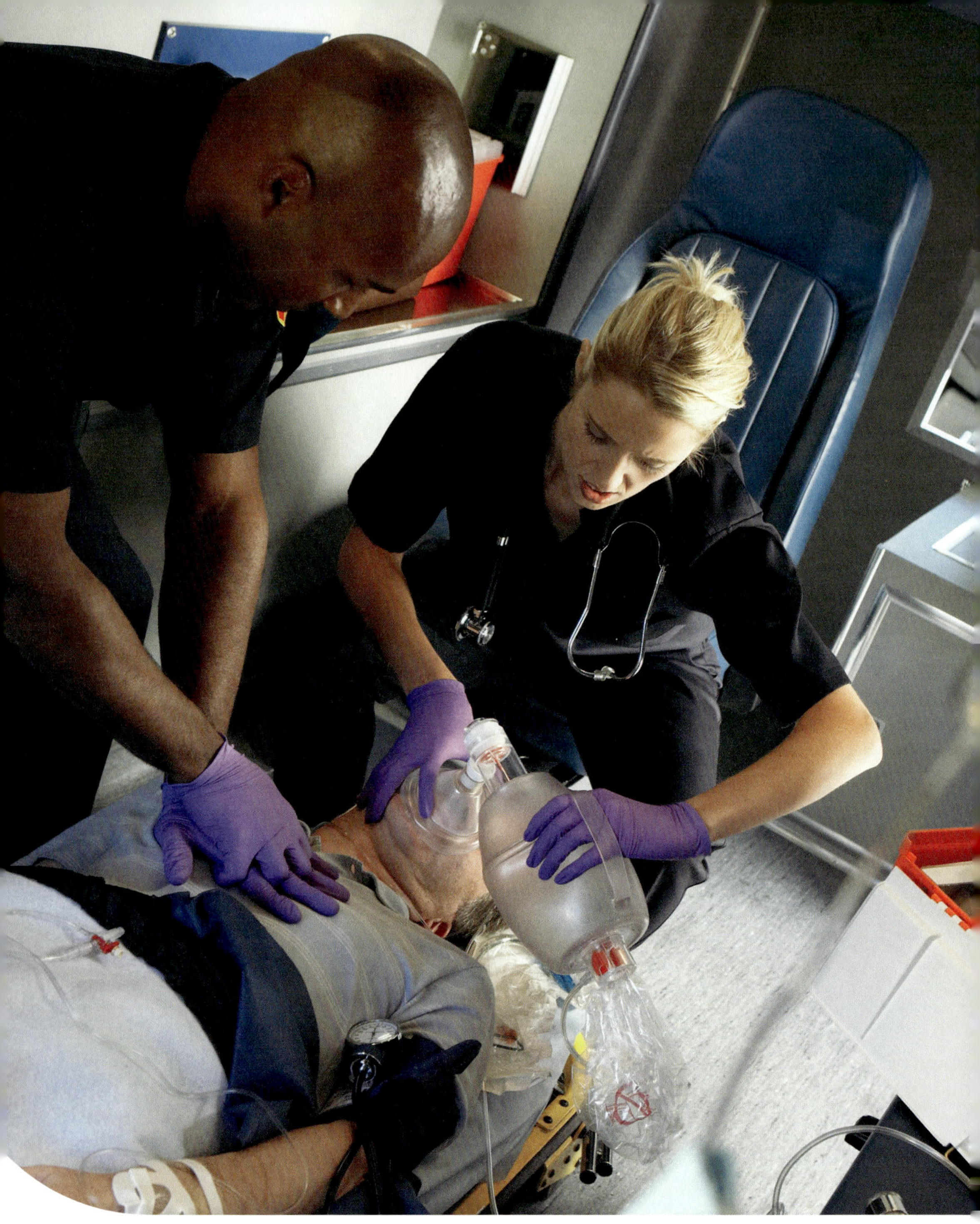

Paramedics transport patients who can't breathe to the
emergency room.

the patient in. Then the emergency room doctor, nurses, and the RT work together. The doctor and nurses treat the injury. The RT makes sure the patient can breathe. The RT also advises the doctor about any breathing issues.

RTs are part of the care team. They examine patients. Therapists also consult with doctors on how to provide breathing care. They help patients breathe. Nurses, medical assistants, and surgeons do their part to improve a patient's health. RTs play a key role on this team. Tara Walker is an RT. "When somebody can't breathe, everyone is calling for you," Walker says. "You're coming in and saving the day."[5]

CHAPTER TWO

WHAT TRAINING DO RESPIRATORY THERAPISTS NEED?

Learning to be an RT is exciting. Students learn skills that will save people's lives. Every RT must graduate from high school. They need to learn basic math and English skills. These skills are important for RTs. Taking more science and math courses is helpful. After high school, students can go to college to study respiratory therapy. There are 2- and 4-year programs.

Students working toward a degree in respiratory therapy balance a mix of classroom and clinical time.

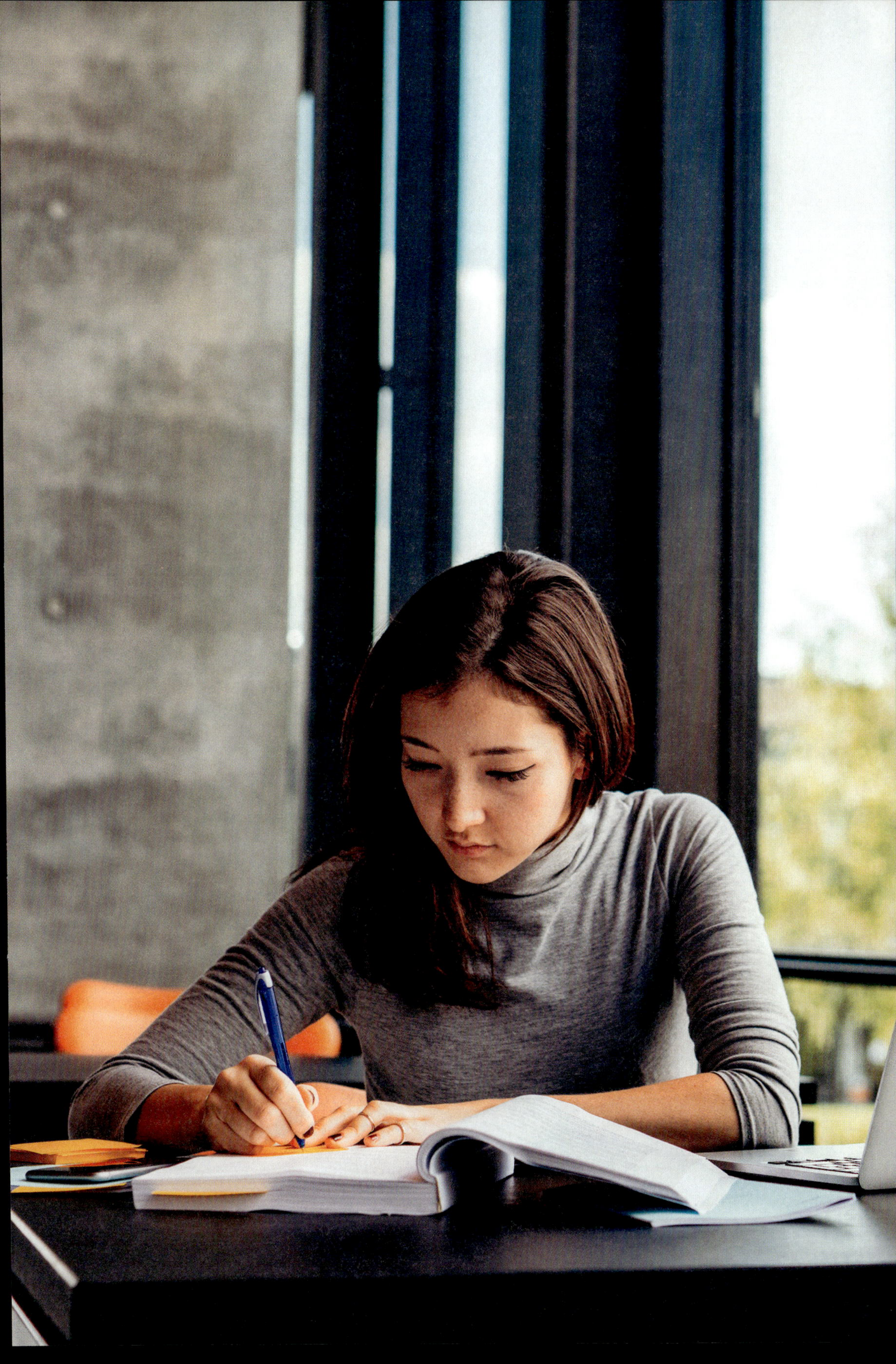

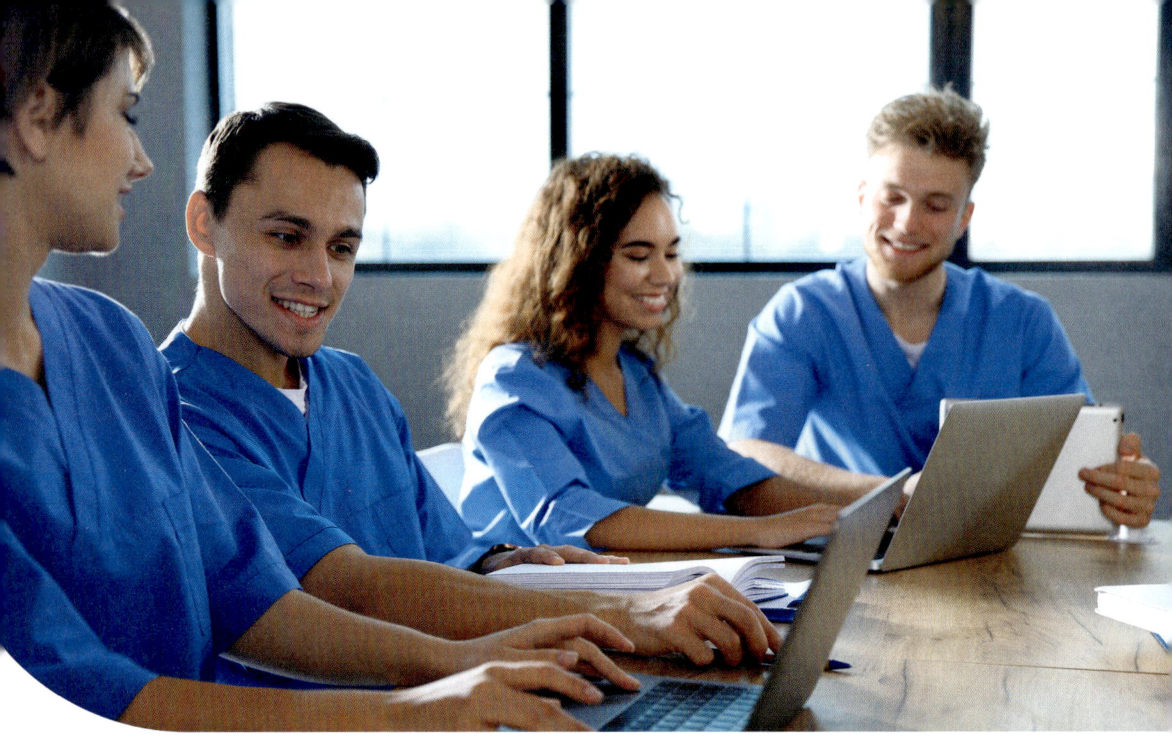

Some students study respiratory therapy for 4 years. They graduate with a bachelor's degree. This degree helps RTs advance to higher positions in the workplace. RTs who want to teach others can continue taking classes to earn a master's degree. This takes a few more years of study. It prepares them to become professors or senior instructors.

ASSOCIATE'S DEGREE

The quickest way to become a respiratory therapist is to get an associate's degree. Some community colleges have respiratory therapy programs. These programs normally take about 3 years. Some colleges are introducing programs that take 2 years. The short programs mean lots of studying. Students should have strong math and science skills.

Education

Seventy-five percent of RTs have a 2-year degree. Fifteen percent have finished their bachelor's degree. The rest have more advanced education. The further RTs advance in school, the easier it is to advance in their careers.

Daytona State College offers a shorter program. "We've just accelerated our program to four semesters," said Misty Carlson. "There's a big need for respiratory therapists and we need to get people out there."[6]

Students learn a lot about the human body. They must understand how the heart and lungs work. They explore how oxygen is moved through the body. Students also learn special medical terms. They learn about drugs that help people breathe. Much of this can be done in the classroom.

SIMULATORS AND LABS

Respiratory therapy also requires hands-on training. Students learn to assess patients. They must figure out how well a person

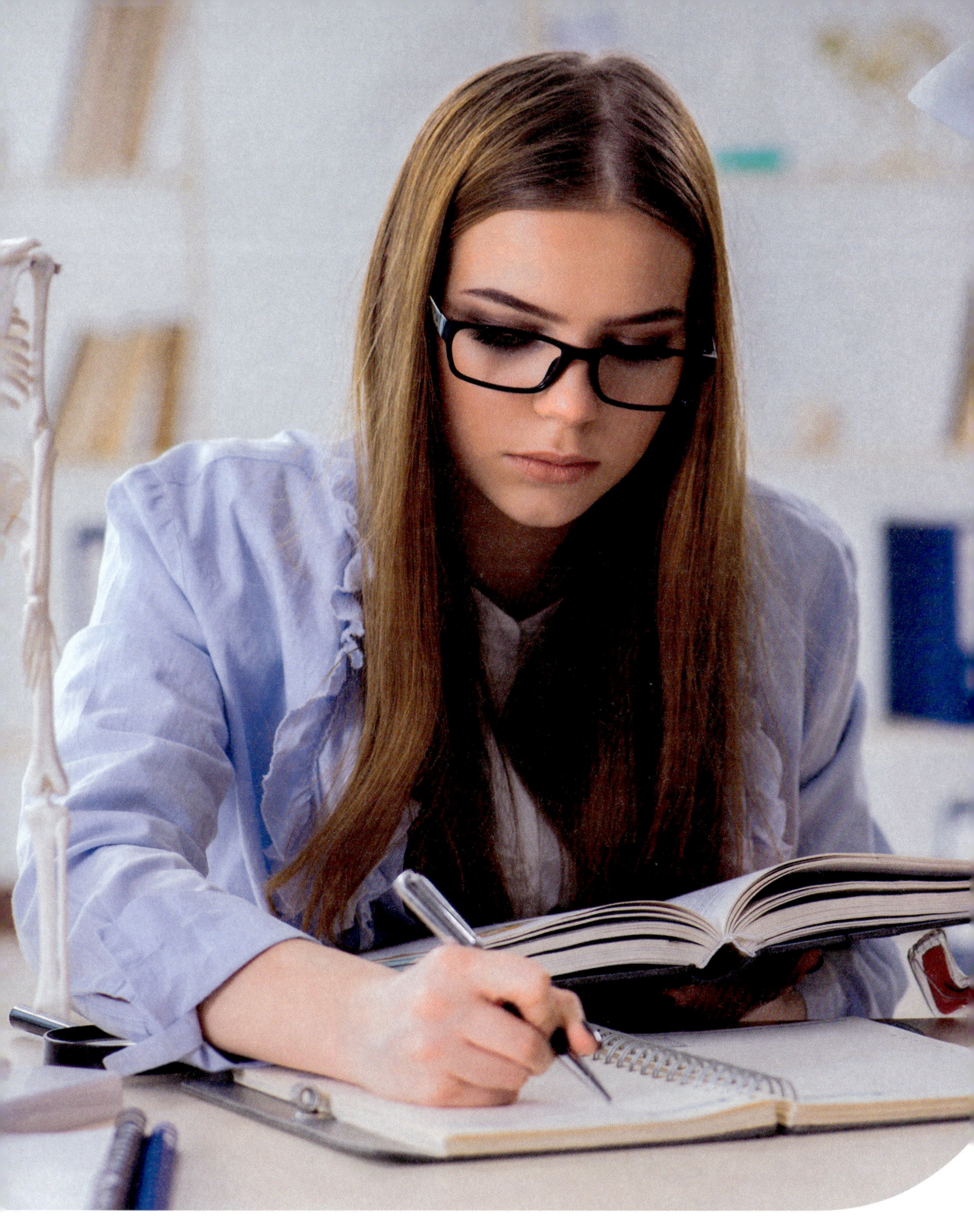

Courses in human anatomy provide an important foundation for those training to be RTs.

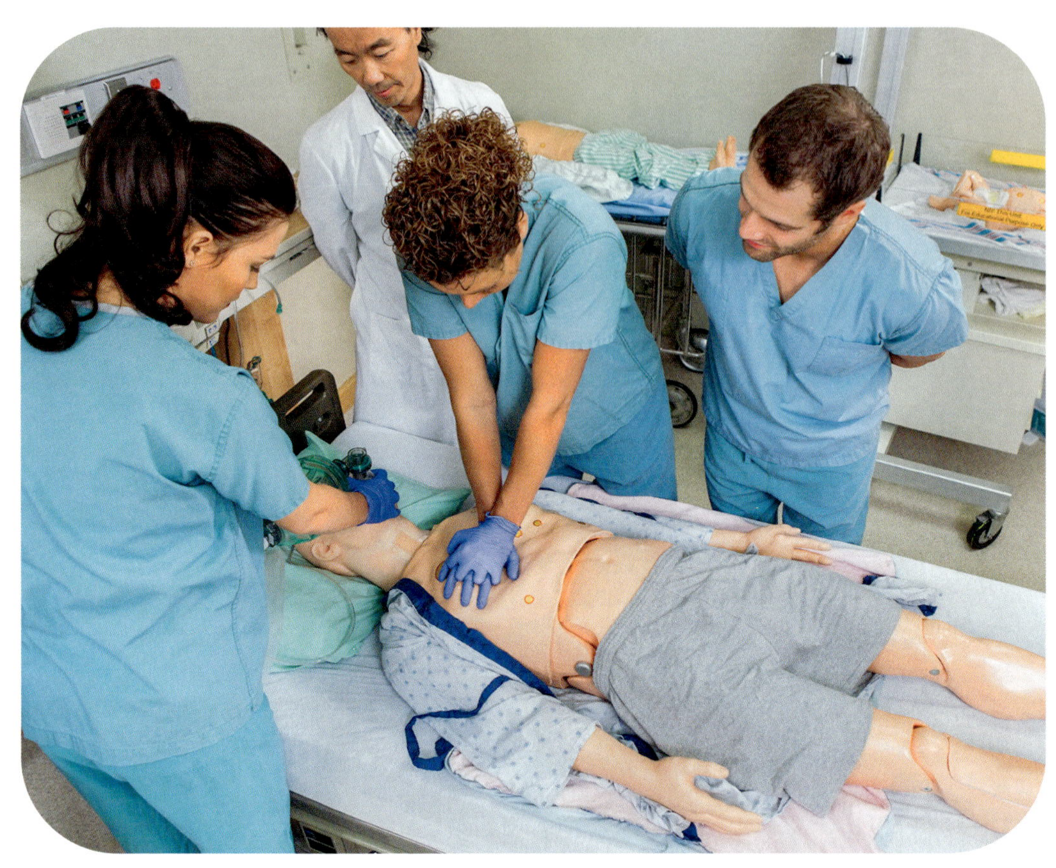

RTs learn by practicing CPR and other skills on a full-size dummy during clinical training.

is breathing. Students also learn how to use a spirometry machine. This measures the air going in and out of a person's lungs. Students practice drawing blood, too.

Some of this practice can be done on other people. But simulators can be used as well. One type of simulator is a fake arm.

The arm has red water pulsing through it. Students use this to practice drawing blood. Another simulator is a full-size adult dummy. Teachers can adjust its breathing and other vital signs. Students practice on the dummy.

Students also practice in actual health care settings. This is called clinical training or a clinical rotation. Students may spend a couple of weeks working in a hospital or clinic. They learn to work as a team with doctors and nurses. They observe and then practice with actual patients. They learn about medications and symptoms. They also learn how to control infections. Students learn how to evaluate a patient's breathing. They learn how to keep a medical chart and take blood pressure. Students help with babies, children, and adults. They assist professional RTs on the job. This provides the students with important real-world experience.

SPECIAL CERTIFICATIONS

Students who graduate can take a test to be officially certified. The test is called the certified respiratory therapist exam. Students who pass the test are officially recognized as certified respiratory therapists (CRTs). Students must have this certification to get a job in every state except Alaska. Some states require a higher certification to get a job. This is called the registered respiratory therapist (RRT) certification. To get this certification, students must pass the CRT exam with a high score. Then they are eligible to take

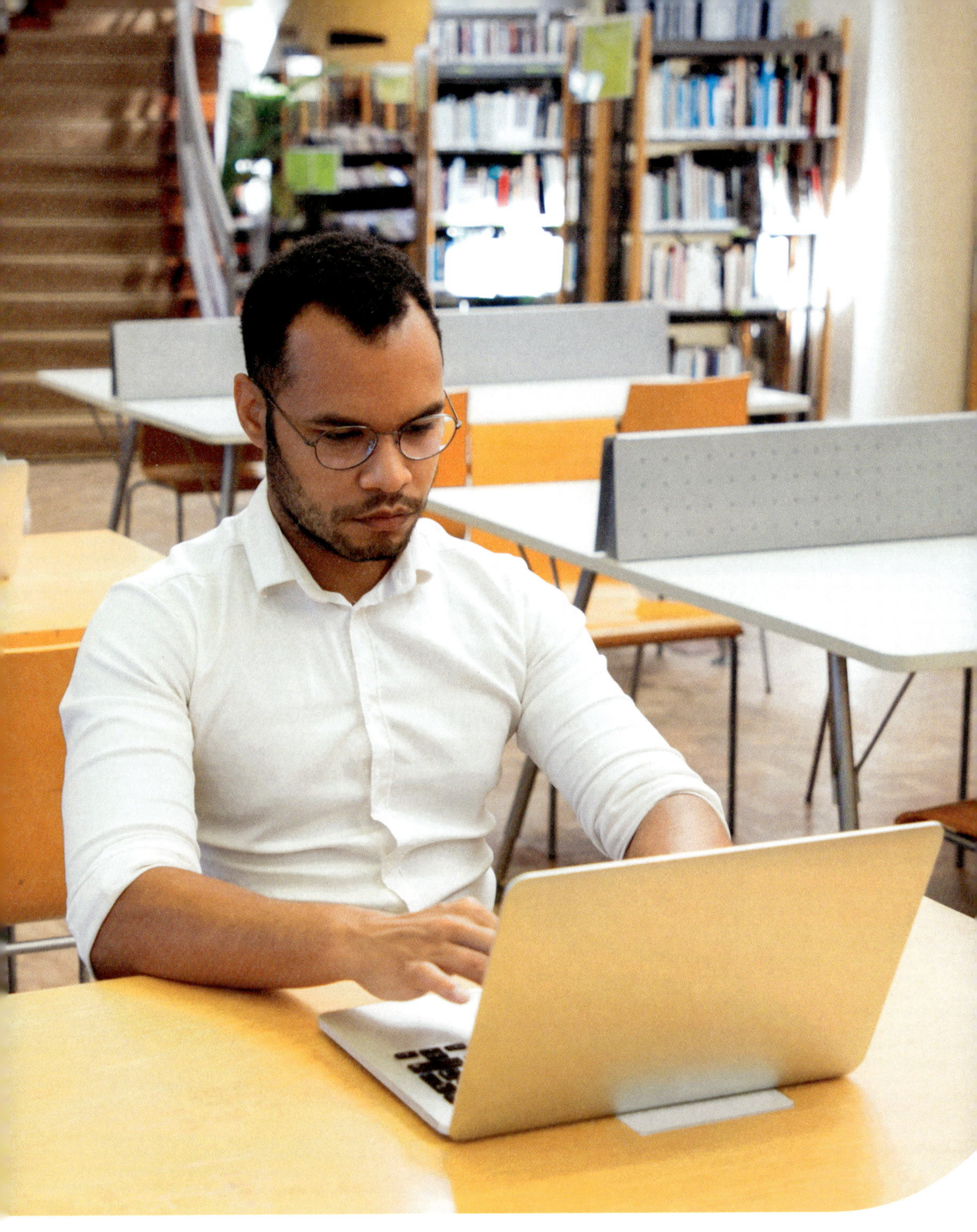

Students must pass a written or online exam to earn CRT certification.

another test. This test is called the clinical simulation evaluation (CSE). Students who pass the CSE are certified as registered respiratory therapists (RRTs). This is a more advanced certification.

Some RTs want to learn even more. They take advanced coursework. These RTs choose from five different types of advanced credentials or specialties. Some learn more about people who have sleep problems. Others specialize in taking care of adults with critical breathing problems. RTs who love working with babies focus on learning how to care for them. There are also special certifications available for heart care and asthma.

Those who finish these programs become experts in their field.

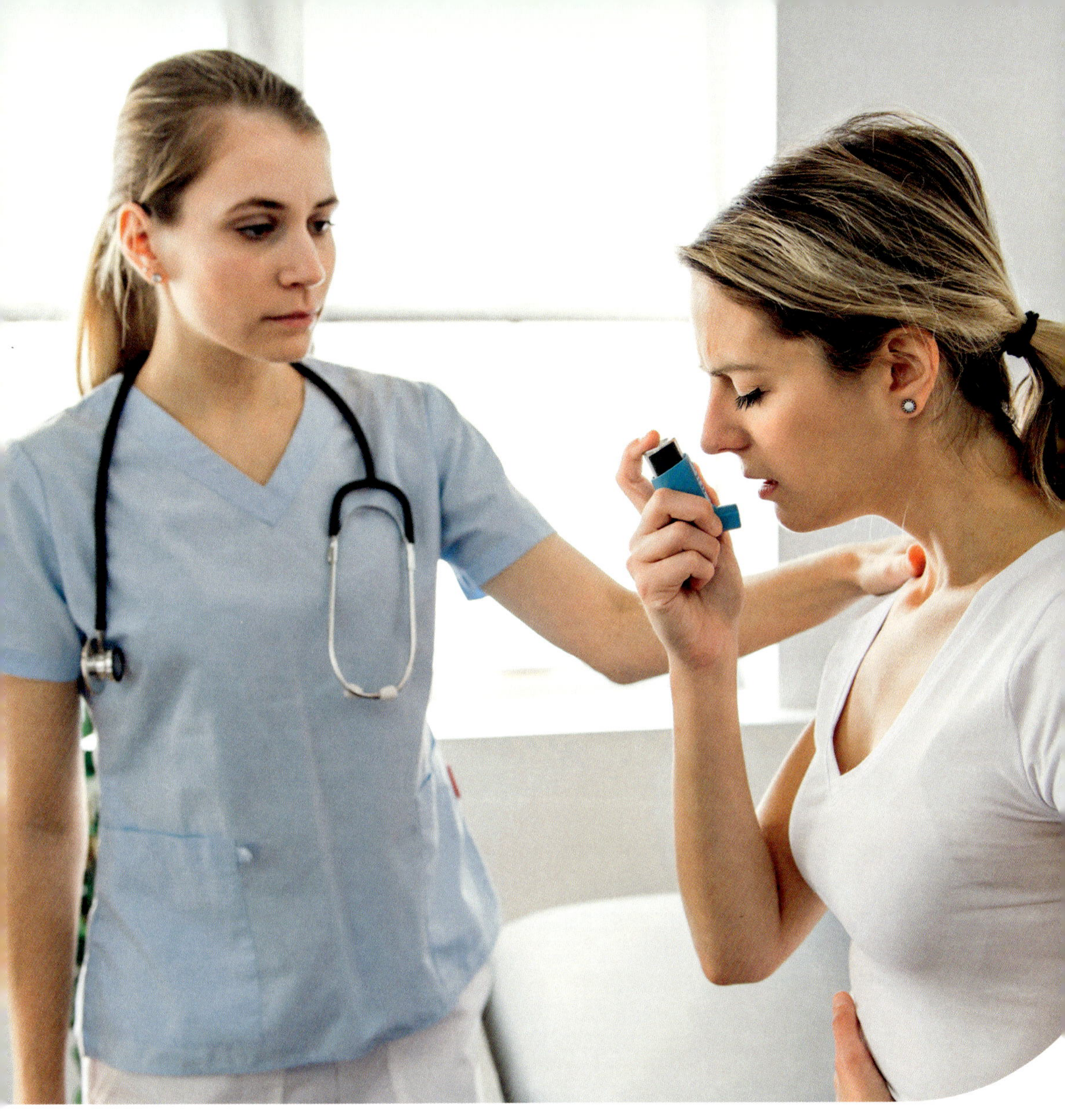

Patients with asthma take medicine through a device called an inhaler.

These specialty credentials make it easier to get a job. They are important for therapists who want to advance in their careers.

WHAT IS LIFE LIKE AS A RESPIRATORY THERAPIST?

Respiratory therapists can choose to work in many varied environments. One RT might work in the emergency room. Another might prefer to transport patients from one place to another. Some choose to work with babies. Others work in sleep centers or heart clinics. RTs with more training are able to take jobs that fit them best.

Some RTs make daily rounds to check in on patients who have respiratory illnesses, including asthma or COVID-19.

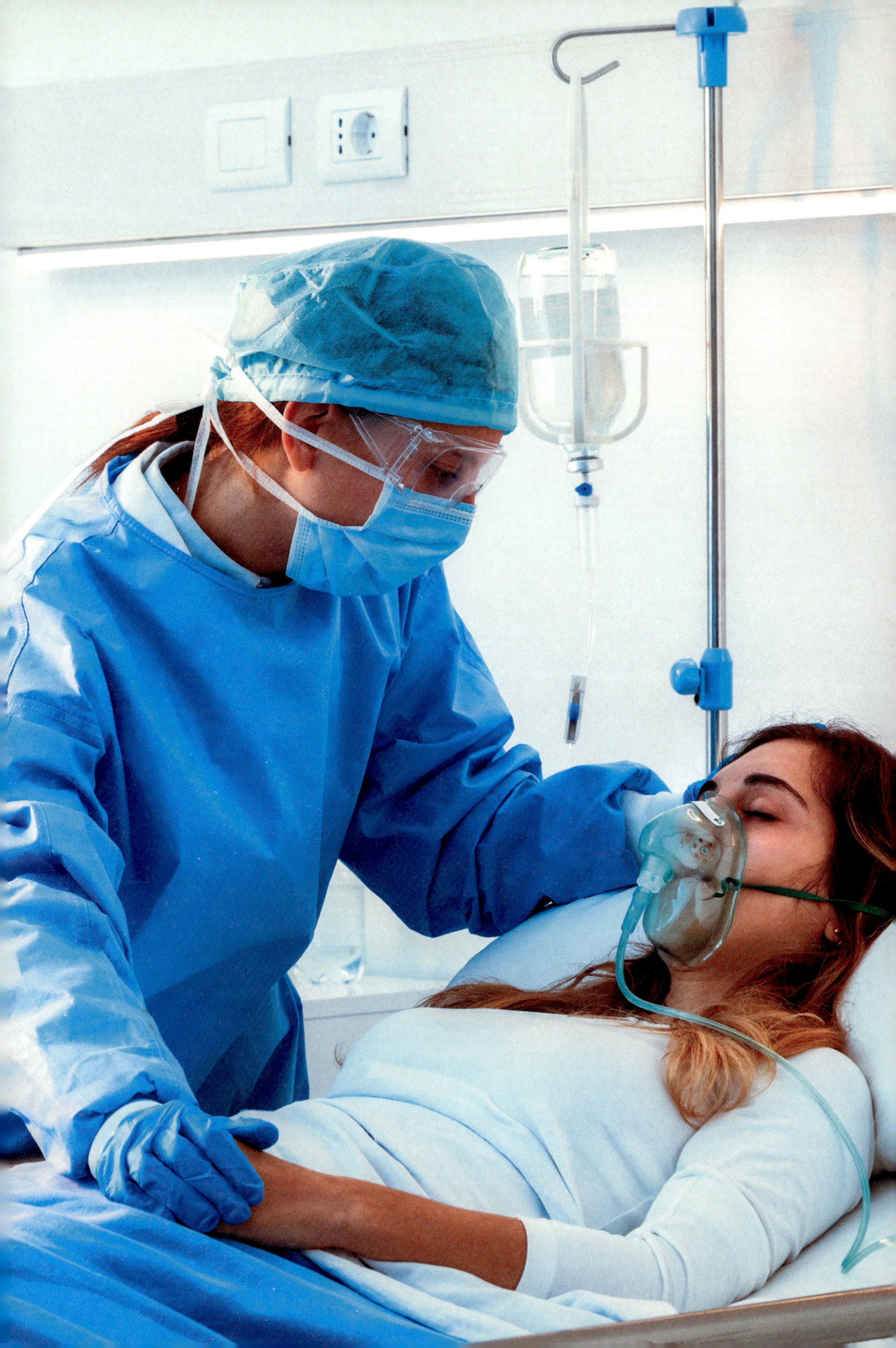

SCHEDULE

Most RTs work in hospitals. Many work a
12-hour schedule. They might start work
at 7:00 a.m. and work all day. Others start
work at 7:00 p.m. and work all night. People
who work the night shift get paid a little
more. Twelve hours of work is a long day.
But full-time therapists can work 3 days a
week and have the other 4 days off.

Respiratory therapists may work in
different units of the hospital. Some
hospitals might assign therapists to a team.
They may work with their team in specific
units in the hospital. Some teams might
work with burn victims. Others may work
with patients who have brain disorders.
Or they might be assigned to work in the
intensive care unit.

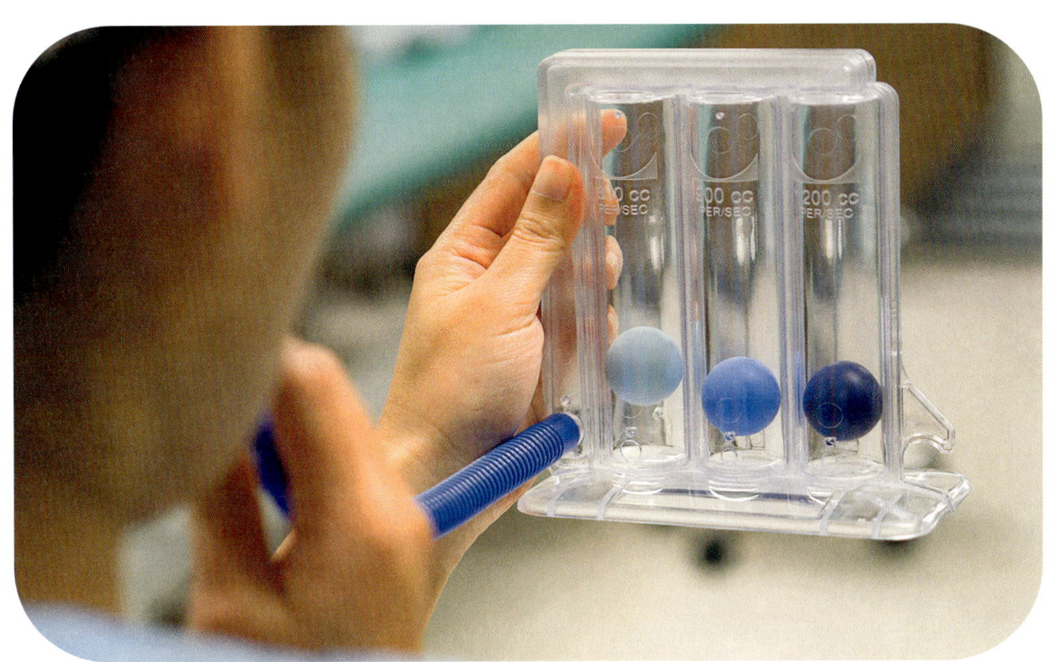

One type of respiratory therapy uses a device called a three-ball spirometer. It helps patients practice deep breathing.

The next week the RT might be doing floor therapy. This is when an RT visits patients who are in the hospital for various reasons. On a typical day, the RTs get a list of patients to see. The patients need breathing treatments. One patient might need a treatment every 2 hours. Another might need treatment every 3 or 4 hours. "We manage the airways and the lungs and

make sure they stay healthy,"[7] explains RT
Katie Lovett. A patient could have asthma
that is getting worse. Another might have a
different breathing problem. RTs usually see
four or five patients each day. RTs work as a
team to care for these patients.

HELPING PEOPLE

RTs introduce themselves to each patient.
They do tests to see how bad a breathing
problem is. They decide how to treat it.
Breathing treatments may involve giving
patients medicine to help them breathe.
The RT sometimes uses a nebulizer to give
the medicine. This is a small device that
changes liquid medicine into a mist. Patients
breathe the mist into their lungs. RTs make
sure the nebulizer is working correctly.

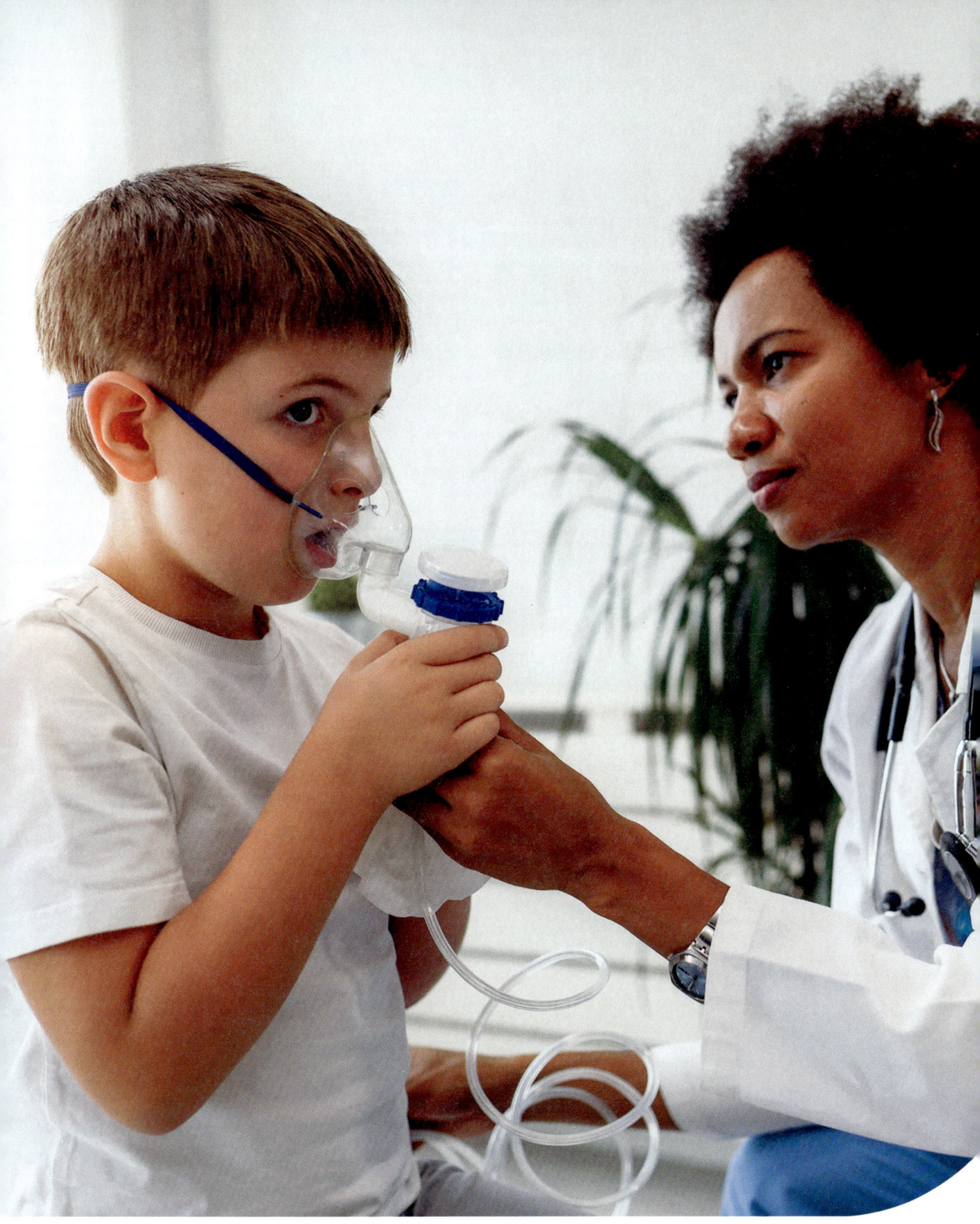

Nebulizers provide an easy way to get medicine into a patient's lungs.

Some patients have mucus in their throats. It blocks their breathing. The therapist uses a **bulb syringe** to suction out the mucus. If there is too much mucus, the RT puts a tube into the patient's throat. The tube is attached to a suction pump machine. The pump pulls out the mucus. The RT stays with each patient for about 30 or 45 minutes.

RTs wear masks while working. Patients can have many kinds of diseases. RTs do

Breathing Medicines

Therapists often use two kinds of medicine to help patients breathe. One type relaxes the muscles in the lungs and opens the airway. Another type reduces swelling. These can be inhaled through a nebulizer.

not want to get sick. When RTs draw blood, they must be extra careful. They do not want to poke themselves with the needle. That is another way they might get sick.

EMERGENCY

Sometimes there is an emergency. Hospitals have special codes for different emergencies. Code blue is an adult medical emergency. Code red means fire. Code white is a **pediatric** emergency. There are several other codes.

When someone has stopped breathing, it is a code blue. The RT quickly grabs the crash cart. The crash cart has important equipment to save people. The therapist and other team members rush to the patient. The RT grabs a bag valve mask.

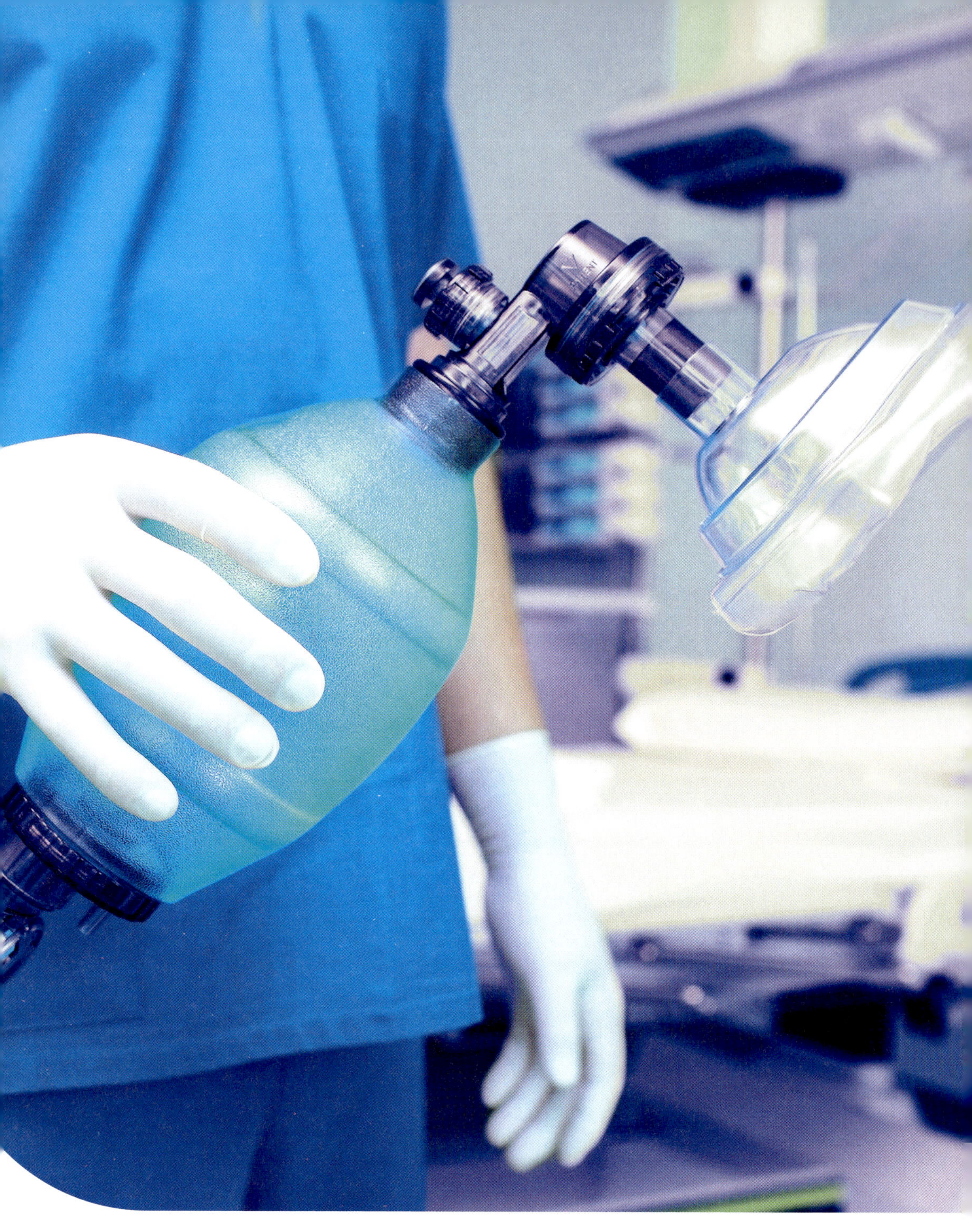

RTs use a device called a bag valve mask to push air into a patient's lungs.

This device looks like a clear football attached to a mask. The RT puts the mask on the patient. They squeeze the football-shaped bag. Each squeeze sends air into the patient's lungs. This helps the patient breathe. Other team members provide assistance as needed. They work together to save the patient.

WHAT IS THE FUTURE FOR RESPIRATORY THERAPISTS?

Respiratory therapists are needed everywhere. Many factors are making breathing problems even worse around the world. These include more smoke from wildfires and pollution from cars and factories. Increasing heat also makes breathing more difficult. Even higher temperatures indoors create issues for those with breathing problems.

Growing environmental risks mean more people are likely to develop breathing issues. RTs will continue to be needed.

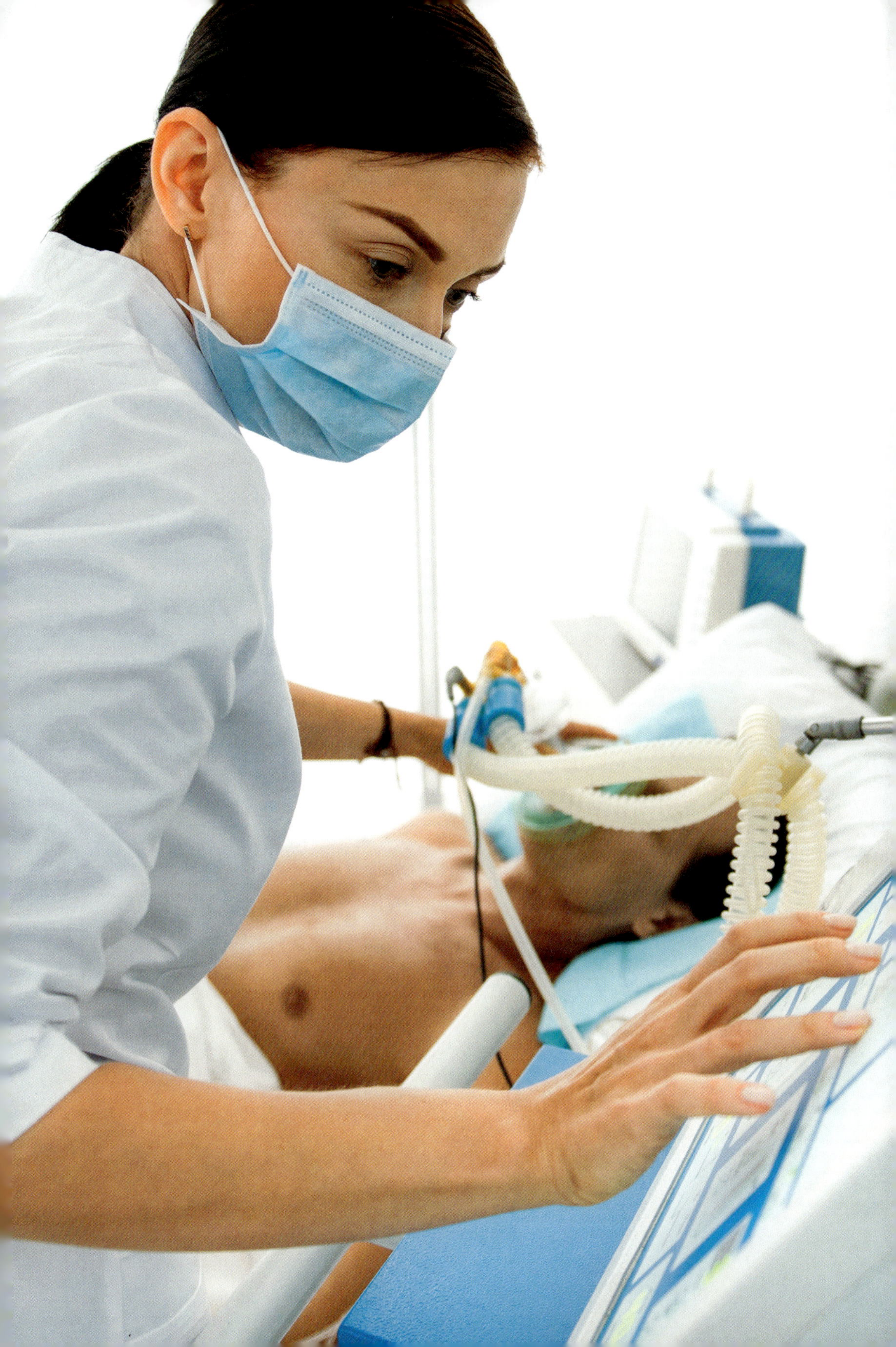

These factors mean the need for new RTs
is increasing.

The US Bureau of Labor Statistics
(BLS) gathers information about different
careers. The news about RTs is promising.
Many new jobs are becoming available.
The BLS expects there to be more than
16,700 new jobs from 2022 to 2032. That is

Other Related Jobs

RTs can do more than work with patients. They
can become instructors in hospitals or professors
at colleges. They can become supervisors.
Therapists can also sell equipment such as
ventilators. Companies need therapists who
know how to use their ventilators. The therapists
are well trained to teach customers how to
use them.

much higher than most other careers.
About 8,600 jobs will become available
every year. Many of these openings are
to replace people who retire or change
occupations. There will be opportunities for
new RTs.

PAY

The average pay for workers in the United
States was about $59,000 in 2023. The
average pay for a registered RT was about
$75,000. That is $16,000 a year more than
the average job.

RTs who become college professors can
make even higher salaries. The average
pay for a college professor in 2023 was
$108,000. Future pay for respiratory
therapists also looks very good. It should

RESPIRATORY THERAPIST MEDIAN WAGES

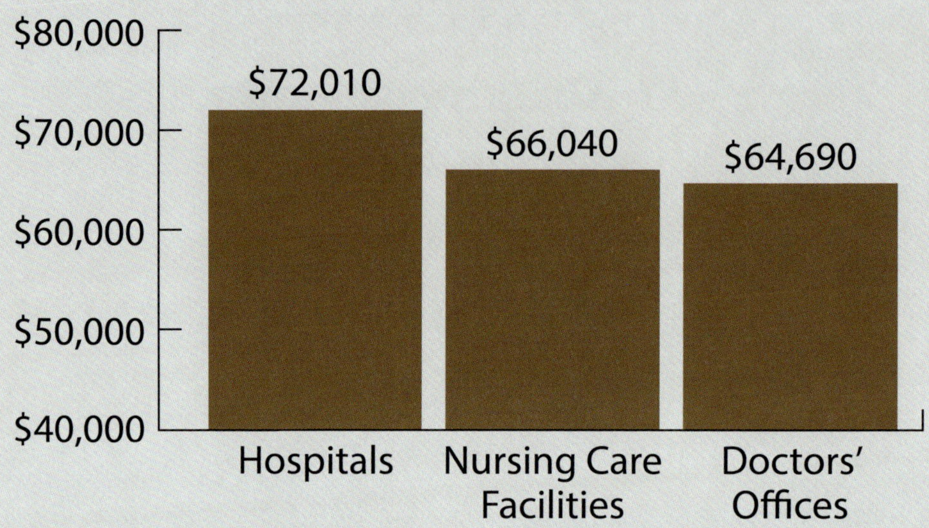

Source: "Respiratory Therapists: Pay," Bureau of Labor Statistics, *September 6, 2023.* www.bls.gov.

The wages for respiratory therapists can vary based on where they work. Here are the median salaries for respiratory therapists in 2022 according to the US Bureau of Labor Statistics.

continue to increase and will remain higher than the average job.

A NEW CAREER PATH

The future of any career always includes change. This is true for RTs. RTs are beginning to take on more responsibility. This is because the number of doctors who take care of heart and breathing problems is declining. This shortage of doctors could reach 12,000 by 2030. With fewer doctors, most hospitals expect RTs to do more. In the past, many RTs were not allowed to put tubes down patients' throats. They could not take arterial blood samples. That has changed.

The American Association for Respiratory Care (AARC) is creating a new career path. It is called advanced practice respiratory therapist (APRT). This career requires a graduate degree in advanced respiratory therapy. An APRT will take on some of the work usually handled by doctors. They will diagnose and treat patients. They can also prescribe some medications. APRTs do work typically done by doctors. Because of this, they are called physician extenders.

TECHNOLOGY

Technology is also changing the field of respiratory therapy. New technology has improved learning in colleges. Many new types of simulators help students learn. These simulators help reduce the amount of staff needed to train students.

RTs use ventilator machines all the time. They are experts in using these machines. There are many different kinds of ventilators. Some add a preset amount of pressure when a patient inhales. Some change the pressure based on how the patient is breathing. Some breathe completely for

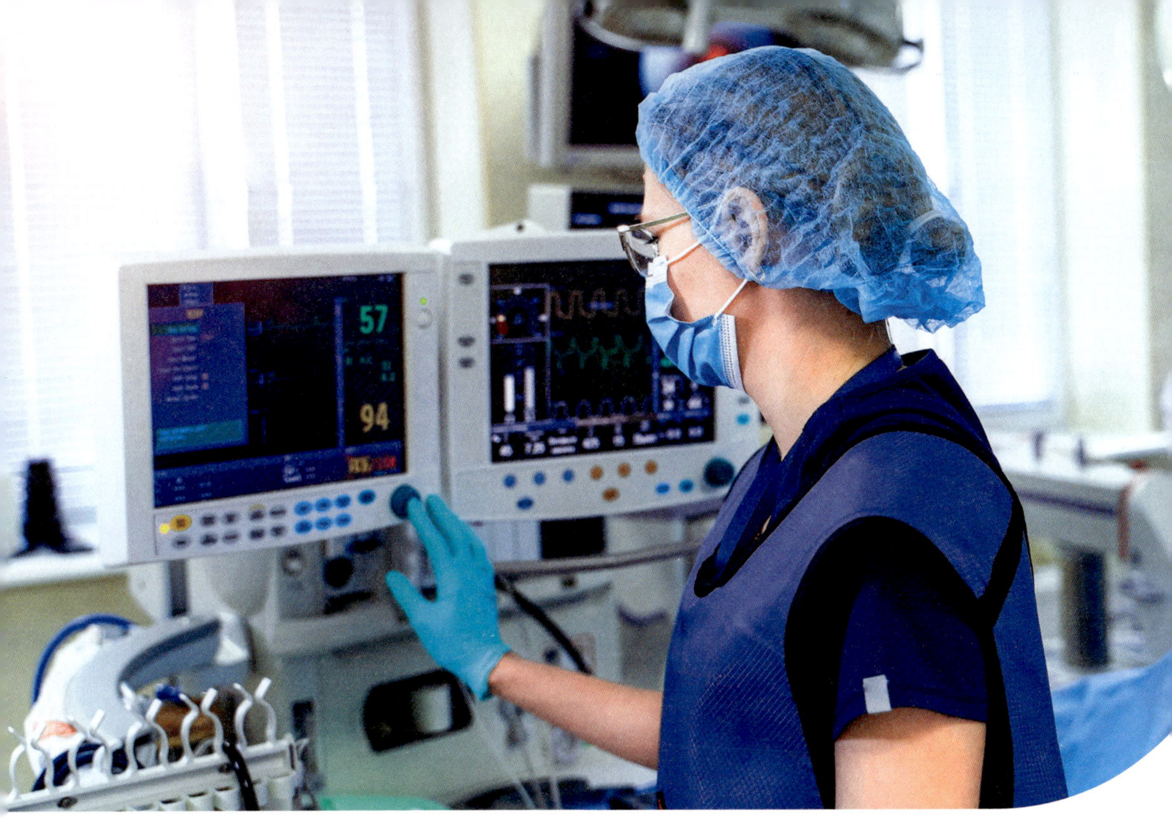

A ventilator monitor displays a patient's heart rate, respiratory rate, blood pressure, and oxygen saturation.

the patient. These can prevent a patient's lungs from collapsing.

RTs know how to use all of these types of machines properly. One exciting new design is a ventilator that can be implanted in the body. It was being tested in early 2023 and will hopefully be available in the future. RTs must keep up with these new advances in technology. They need to know how to work all kinds of ventilators and fix any problems. This requires study and training.

THE WORKFORCE

Respiratory therapy is not a very diverse field. About 63.5 percent of respiratory therapists are white. Hispanic people make up 14.6 percent. About 11 percent are Black, and 6.4 percent are Asian. About 62.5 percent of RTs are women. Around 9 percent of RTs are in the LGBTQ community.

There are challenges in the respiratory therapy field. Female therapists are often not paid as much as men. Female RTs average about 7 percent lower pay than

men in the field. Another challenge can be
the long hours many RTs work. Working
a few 12-hour shifts in a row can be very
tiring. And, in some cases, the job requires

While the days can be long, the ability to help patients breathe makes respiratory therapy a satisfying career.

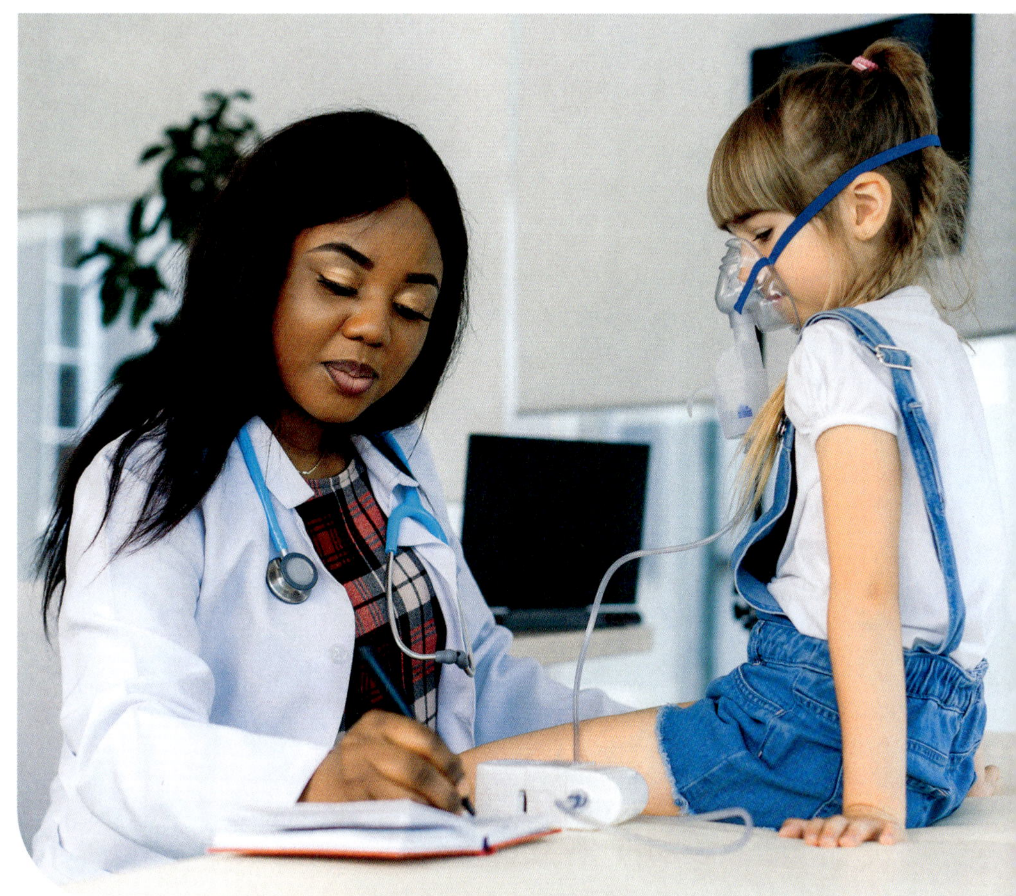

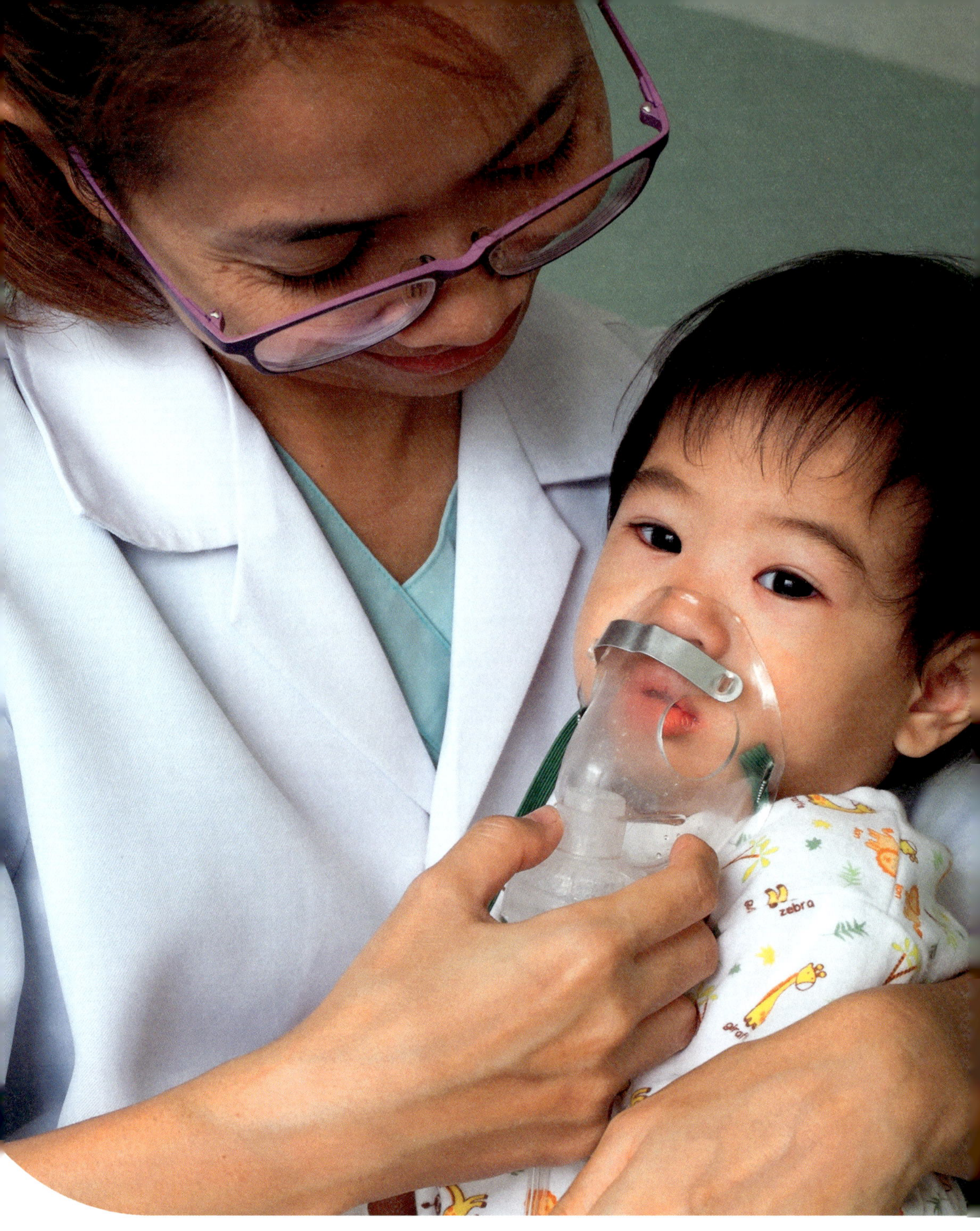

Helping babies breathe comfortably is a rewarding part
of the job for many respiratory therapists.

therapists to lift heavy oxygen bottles. This can be difficult for some people.

But for many, it is a rewarding career. RT Beth Howell explained what she likes about her job. "If you want to be part of every single bit of health care," said Howell, "respiratory is the way to go. Because you can pick what you want to do. You get to specialize in everything. . . . There is only one department required in every single, solitary life support code, and that is a respiratory therapist."[8]

GLOSSARY

bulb syringe

a bulb with a narrow tube used to suction out mucus

COPD

chronic obstructive pulmonary disease, a condition that makes it hard to breathe

CPAP machine

continuous positive airway pressure machine, a device that helps people breathe

critical care patients

patients with life-threatening problems or diseases

micro preemies

babies born before 26 weeks of gestation

mucus

a thick, slippery liquid found in the nose, mouth, throat, and lungs

neonatal

relating to newborn babies

pediatric

a branch of medicine that involves caring for children

pneumonia

a lung infection that can make it hard to breathe

SOURCE NOTES

INTRODUCTION: WHY BECOME A RESPIRATORY THERAPIST?

1. Misty Carlson, Personal interview, August 18, 2023.

2. Misty Carlson, Personal interview, August 18, 2023.

CHAPTER ONE: WHAT DOES A RESPIRATORY THERAPIST DO?

3. Gina Ricard, Personal interview, August 18, 2023.

4. Beth Howell, Personal interview, August 21, 2023.

5. Tara Walker, Personal interview, August 15, 2023.

CHAPTER TWO: WHAT TRAINING DO RESPIRATORY THERAPISTS NEED?

6. Misty Carlson, Personal interview, August 18, 2023.

CHAPTER THREE: WHAT IS LIFE LIKE AS A RESPIRATORY THERAPIST?

7. Quoted in "A Day in the Life: Respiratory Therapist," Cincinnati Children's, *YouTube*, April 5, 2021. www.youtube.com.

CHAPTER FOUR: WHAT IS THE FUTURE FOR RESPIRATORY THERAPISTS?

8. Beth Howell, Personal interview, August 21, 2023.

FOR FURTHER RESEARCH

BOOKS

Kerry Dinmont, *Frontline Workers During Covid-19*. San Diego, CA: BrightPoint Press, 2021.

Professor Alice Roberts, *The Complete Human Body*. New York: DK Publishing, 2023.

Marne Ventura, *Become a Licensed Practical Nurse*. San Diego, CA: BrightPoint Press, 2025.

INTERNET SOURCES

"How Lungs Work," *American Lung Association*, September 29, 2023. www.lung.org.

"Respiratory Therapy: Essential Care for Kids with Breathing Woes," *Children's Hospital of Richmond*, October 25, 2021. www.chrichmond.org.

"What Is Asthma?," *Nemours Teens Health*, September 2023. www.kidshealth.org.

WEBSITES

Asthma
www.kidshealth.org/en/teens/asthma

The Nemours Teens Health website explains what asthma is and answers frequently asked questions. It also provides tips for how to manage asthma triggered by different environmental causes.

Be An RT
www.be-an-rt.org

The Be An RT website provides an overview of the profession. It also includes detailed steps for how to become a respiratory therapist, including what classes to take in high school.

Minnesota Pollution Control Agency: Air Quality and Health
www.pca.state.mn.us

The Minnesota Pollution Control Agency website shows how pollution affects people. It discusses different types of pollution and the physical problems they cause.

INDEX

IMAGE CREDITS

Cover: © Visivasnc/iStockphoto

5: © Microgen/Shutterstock Images

7: © Zhuravlev Andrey/Shutterstock Images

9: © chalermphon_tiam/Shutterstock Images

11: © Joa Souza/Shutterstock Images

13: © Lorenzo Photo Projects/Shutterstock Images

15: © Studio13lights/Shutterstock Images

17: © Terelyuk/Shutterstock Images

20: © Juice Verve/Shutterstock Images

22: © Monkey Business Images/Shutterstock Images

25: © Jacob Lund/Shutterstock Images

26: © New Africa/Shutterstock Images

29: © Elnur/Shutterstock Images

30: © Tyler Olson/Shutterstock Images

33: © Mangostar/Shutterstock Images

35: © Lopolo/Shutterstock Images

37: © alessandro guerriero/Shutterstock Images

39: © nuiza11/Shutterstock Images

41: © Lordn/Shutterstock Images

44: © sfam_photo/Shutterstock Images

47: © Olena Yakobchuk/Shutterstock Images

50: © Red Line Editorial

53: © Terelyuk/Shutterstock Images

55: © SofikoS/Shutterstock Images

56: © donghero/Shutterstock Images

ABOUT THE AUTHOR

Mike Downs is the author of more than thirty books for young people. He loves writing books that kids are excited to read. Mike has written fiction (fantasy, memoir, and poetry) and nonfiction (geography, aerospace, and science). A couple of his books are *The Flying Man: Otto Lilienthal, The World's First Pilot* and *A Treasure of Measures*.